How My Husband and I Survived his Stroke

How My Husband and I Survived his Stroke

W. F. ROWAN

Copyright © 2023 W. F. Rowan

This work is copyright. Apart from any fair dealing for the purposes of private study, research, criticism or review, as permitted by the Copyright Act 1968, no part of this book may be reproduced, stored in a retrieval system or transmitted in any form or by any means, electronic, mechanical, photocopying, recording or otherwise, without the prior written permission of the publisher.

W. F. Rowan — How my Husband and I Survived His Stroke

ISBN 978-0-6456123-4-9 (paperback)

A catalogue record for this book is available from the National Library of Australia

Editing: Kristina Proft
Cover and internal design: Ronald Proft
Delphian Books
Unit 1, 29 Mile End Road, Rouse Hills, NSW 2155
delphianbooks.com.au
Cover graphic: Original image (Pixabay)

Disclaimer: Although the author and publisher have made every effort to ensure that the information in this book was correct at press time, the author and publisher do not assume and hereby disclaim any liability to any party for any loss, damage, or disruption caused by errors or omissions, whether such errors or omissions result from negligence, accident, or any other cause.

This book is autobiographical and is not intended as a means of disseminating medical advice. Content contained in or accessed through the book should not be relied upon for medical purposes in any way. The advice of a medical practitioner should always be obtained.

Contents

Preface	vii
Introduction	1
What is a stroke and what causes it?	1
Who is at risk of stroke?	1
Some symptoms of stroke	2
Chapter 1 Our world falls apart	3
What happened and why?	4
Seeking help: physiotherapy	8
Further help: the GP	9
Westmead Hospital	10
Chapter 2 Picking up the pieces	15
An important birthday, in more ways than one	15
Permission to travel	16
A work opportunity	18
Chapter 3 Presenting symptoms: Memory, Fatigue, Anger and Depression	21
Memory	21
Fatigue	23
Medications and their side effects	25
Navigating the depression and anger	31
The things that helped	32
The things that didn't help	33
Tinnitus	34
Dizziness/Balance	37
The darkest times	38
Chapter 4 Friendships	39
Chapter 5 Moving forward some more	42
The 15-year mark	43
The SES	44
What now?	45
Chapter 6 Things I have learned	48
Do you have a will?	48
Do you have life insurance?	48
Afterword	50
Support	51
Do you, or does someone you know, need help?	51

Special Thanks

To Christine for your support on the fateful day.

Neil B who, knowing of Peter's condition, helped with employment in the early stages which kept us afloat whilst we adjusted to our new reality.

Howard – who provided Peter some paid work he could do from home, and still does to this day.

Dave, our brother from another mother. Your love and support is immeasurable and has kept us both from slipping into despair.

Our dogs, past and present for your constant love and affection.

For all the 'good and positive' who remained in our lives.

Finally, for Nicole who sparked the idea for pen to paper.

Preface

To remain indifferent to the challenges we face is indefensible. If the goal is noble, whether or not it is realized within our lifetime is largely irrelevant. What we must do, therefore, is to strive, and persevere, and never give up.

DALAI LAMA XIV

I wrote this book in the hope that it will help people navigate the emotional trauma caused by having a stroke and some of the side effects that may present themselves.

Although we did seek legal advice with what happened to Peter, I am not going to go into that part of our story simply because everyone is different, has a different story and quite frankly I am not in a position to tell people if they should or shouldn't seek legal advice. If in doubt, talk to your trusted professional.

I will go into some detail about how Peter came to have a stroke, and deeper details on the side effects he suffered as a result of that and what we did individually and as a family to manage the ramifications. Although I have not discussed the legal path we took or our financial situation before, during, or after we did learn very quickly how to manage our finances a lot better.

One thing I will stress here – Don't hesitate. If there is a medical issue, call for help immediately.

W. F. Rowan
July 2023

Introduction

What is a stroke and what causes it?

Briefly, a stroke is a medical emergency where blood flow to the brain is reduced and the brain is deprived of oxygen. If this happens, brain cells will begin to die.

The disruption of blood can happen in two ways:

1. an *ischaemic stroke,* where the obstruction of blood is caused by an embolism or thrombus (blood clot) within the blood vessel coming loose and travelling from one part of the body to the brain; this type of stroke can also be caused by a narrowing of the arteries (stenosis). A transient ischaemic attack (TIA) is a temporary version of this, sometimes known as a mini stroke, which (generally) leaves no lasting symptoms
2. a *haemorrhagic stroke,* where there is bleeding in the brain following an artery breaking open or leaking blood. The bleeding creates excess pressure in the skull and swells the brain, causing damage to brain cells and tissue.

Who is at risk of stroke?

Risk factors could include:
- Being overweight
- Having a sedentary life
- Binge drinking
- Diabetes
- Smoking
- High blood pressure

- High cholesterol
- Family history of stroke
- Cardiovascular diseases
- Age – people above age 55 are at higher risk
- Gender – men are considered to be at higher risk of stroke than women

The above are classic risk factors for a stroke. It should be noted that other forms of injury could also trigger a stroke – a vehicle accident (whiplash) or blunt force trauma, just as an example. The above list should not be taken as definitive, as other situations could also cause a stroke.

Some symptoms of stroke

Some stroke symptoms that may present themselves are:
- Face (drooping on one side)
- Arms (unable to lift)
- Speech (slurred)
- Intense Headache (migraine level)
- Dizziness
- Nausea
- Cold Sweats

Symptoms may vary from person to person, depending on the type of stroke suffered and not all symptoms are visible.

Note: The details above have been sourced from a number of online sites and are for informational purposes only. Consult a medical professional for advice on your own condition.

CHAPTER 1

Our world falls apart

Courage is grace under pressure
ERNEST HEMINGWAY

Early August 2004, just a few weeks short of my husband's 40th birthday, our world came to an abrupt halt.

From minor muscular pain requiring massage to a massive brain injury.

There are many holes in my memory now, but some things are as clear as if they happened only last week. At the time adrenaline kicked in and shock hit the system. It is only now, 19 years later, that the trauma has subsided to the point that I can put pen to paper and I can share the experience in the hope that it may help others – individuals and families – to navigate what they could possibly expect from such an event. I say family, because it is not only the victim of stroke who is affected. Children, partners and friends all have a part to play. It still moves me to tears at times when I think of everything we lost, but I also remind myself quite often that we didn't lose everything. *My husband is still with me.*

There is so much more help available these days that we simply didn't either know about or had access to back then. If it was available, no one really sat down and told us about it. For the most part we fumbled along. Thankfully we had tremendous support from some very close friends. And to be blunt, without them I doubt both of us, or at least one of us, would have made it this far. The doctors and our neurology professor were great, don't get me wrong, but there is quite a difference between visiting a professional office, then going home to your everyday life. The understanding and support from friends was probably more vital than family. I will cover off more on this a little later.

What happened and why?

It started with some shoulder pain – possibly from doing too much gardening but could have been anything, because you know, when you are young and fit, you feel invincible. Our physiotherapist was away on holidays so, for the first time in Peter's life, we went to a chiropractor. We went to him because his daughter and ours went to school together and for no other reason. Doing our bit to keep business within the circle as such. Our daughter and his were not exceedingly close, but they lived fairly close to us and on occasion we carpooled when there were sporting events, school transport issues, or exams at odd times (our girls were in senior high school).

Upon arrival at the clinic, the chiropractor did some remedial massage around the pained area. I don't recall Peter ever being asked to lay down and from my memory, he was in a seated position for the duration of the appointment. The chiropractor had Peter sit up straight as he positioned himself to do a fast neck manipulation procedure. He placed his hands on either side of Peter's head and neck and twisted his head, with one swift movement from left to right.

But here is one detail I remember very distinctly: At the exact moment this procedure was performed, Peter turned to me and stated 'Geeze, that was hot.' He had felt a searing pain, like heat, on the left side of his neck. It was later thought that the placement of the chiropractor's thumb just happened to press and pinch exactly on his carotid artery *(see Diagram 1)* and during the twist it was stretched causing a 9-centimetre tear on the inner lining of the artery.

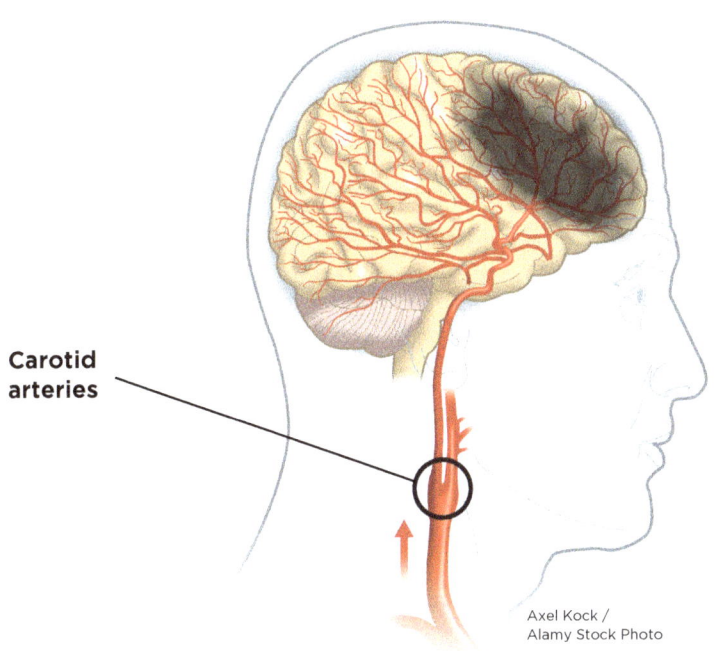

Axel Kock / Alamy Stock Photo

Diagram 1: Carotid arteries
Carotid arteries are major blood vessels in the neck that supply blood to the brain, face and neck.

We didn't think any more about it at that time – at least not for a couple of weeks. We do not recall the fast neck manipulation being explained to Peter and we were not asked if Peter consented to this procedure. Nor were we advised of any possible risks associated with the procedure. As we had never been to a chiropractor before, we didn't know what to expect or if there was any process that had to be followed. It is also possible that the familiarity played a part, from the chiropractor's point of view that is. Who knows, and there is no way to verify that detail now.

Fast forward a couple of weeks. Peter was working with our neighbour in a warehouse helping install dust extraction systems. They usually started work at around 7 am and had a morning break at around 9 am. The required WHS (Work, Health and Safety) equipment – eye protection and hard hat – were worn at all times on site. Just before morning break, Peter bent over to pick up a tool and very lightly bumped his hard hat rim on the wall.

This was the 'crunch' point. What we didn't realise, at the time, was that the chiropractor, at the moment of doing the fast neck manipulation, stretched the main artery on the left side of Peter's neck, resulting in the inner lining of the artery tearing – a tear of approximately 9 centimetres. During those past couple of weeks, a 'scab' of cells had built up in this area and the slight jarring of the hard hat on the wall dislodged this 'scab' as a clot. It travelled to the thalamus *(see Diagram 2)* part of his brain, causing a stroke.

It was that simple and that dramatic.

Little did we know at any time during this just what an impact it would have on our whole lives.

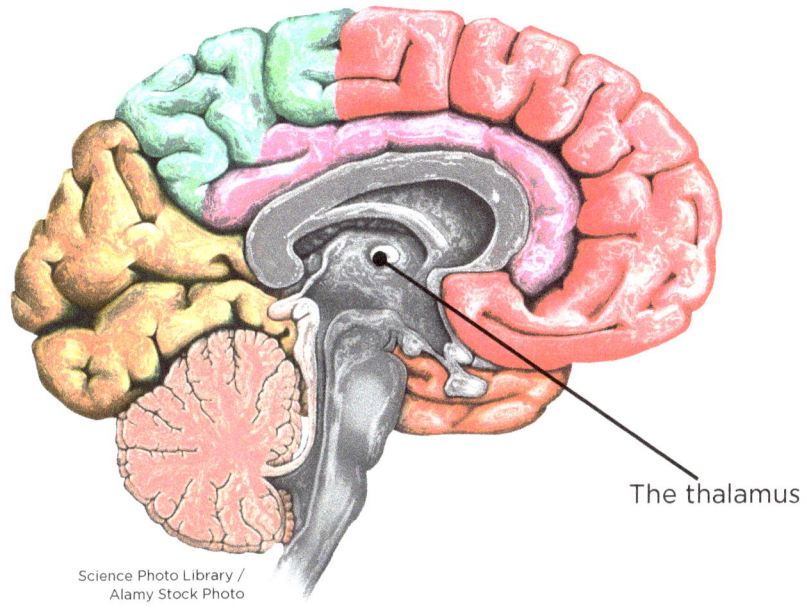

Science Photo Library / Alamy Stock Photo

The thalamus

Diagram 2: The thalamus

The thalamus, situated at the top of the brain stem, relays information to related areas in the cerebral cortex so that the following roles are performed:

- Information from all the senses (taste, touch, hearing, seeing), except smell, are transmitted
- Motor (movement) information is relayed to motor pathways.
- Prioritizing attention. The thalamus helps decide what to focus on among the vast amount of information that it receives
- Consciousness. The thalamus contributes to perception and plays a role in sleep and wakefulness
- Thinking (cognition) and memory

The thalamus is connected with structures of the limbic system, which is involved in processing and regulating emotions, formation and storage of memories, sexual arousal and learning.

When Peter walked into the lunchroom (within minutes of the hard hat knock), his colleagues commented how pale he was looking. Peter stated he has just had a massive migraine start. It was not uncommon for Peter to have headaches – many years of looking at computer screens (he had previously worked in IT) can certainly strain the eyes. But clearly this was more than a headache. It was suggested to him that an ambulance be called. But back then, Peter was the type of male to say, 'Nope, don't need an ambulance, I can drive, I'll be right, I'll just go home.'

In hindsight, we should have called an ambulance regardless. Thinking back on this now and knowing how long it was between the injury and Peter getting to hospital, we are so lucky not to have lost him.

Seeking help: physiotherapy

Peter did call me just before he left to go home, asking me to make an appointment (this time) with the physio so he could get some remedial massage to hopefully ease the migraine. I recall it was around early to mid afternoon when we got to the physiotherapist's office. Peter had been asleep on our bed for a few hours before I got home to take him to the physio. He could just as easily have slipped into a coma and died.

The next thing Peter remembered was me waking him up to take him to the physio office. To this day, Peter has no recollection of how he managed to drive home from Bankstown to Rouse Hill. For some weeks I had expected him to receive a fine for running a red light, or for speeding, but nothing came. I guess working on Auto Pilot is a real thing!

Our physio – Philip Wood Physiotherapy – had his practice fairly close by in Riverstone – about 20 minutes' drive from home. At this time, we were still of the assumption that Peter was suffering a massive migraine. He was to some degree, but the pain was just somewhat more severe and intense than we had realised.

Peter hadn't even been receiving treatment for 5 minutes before the physiotherapist came rushing out to open doors and clear a path for Peter to go to the bathroom. He stumbled out and proceeded to hug the toilet bowl for about 15 to 20 minutes. He didn't throw up but was in a constant state of feeling like he wanted to. An ambulance was once again mentioned; however, I bundled Peter into the car (with a bucket, just in case) and headed off immediately to our GP's office.

Philip Wood's physiotherapy notes from Peter's visit

Further help: the GP

At this time, and even today, Peter cannot recall these immediate events. However, he had one small window of clarity when we reached the doctor's surgery, where they provided him with some oxygen. Their comment was they simply did not have the equipment on hand to deal with whatever was happening to him and they said he needed to go to hospital. So off we went again heading toward Westmead. Another missed opportunity to call an ambulance.

Westmead Hospital

I honestly cannot remember how I was personally feeling at this time. I'm sure some panic was beginning to creep in, because I called one of my friends who had previously been a nurse and asked her to come down to the hospital. At a subconscious level, I knew I needed someone there with me for support and who could think clearly. By this time, Peter had had his stroke approximately mid-morning, and we were on the way to the hospital in the mid to late afternoon. The only relief he had received was a few minutes of oxygen given at the GP's surgery. In hindsight, this one small act – receiving a burst of oxygen – may have been enough to reduce the overall impact of the stroke. I hate to think how much worse it could have been otherwise.

Peter wasn't admitted to a bed at the hospital until the evening – I think at around 9 pm. One of the initial tests was a lumbar puncture *(see Diagram 3)* (Peter remembers this being quite painful), then they carried out an MRI (magnetic resonance imaging). This clearly showed where the injury was and showed he had suffered a Transient Ischaemic Attack (TIA). Having the MRI done was vital to our future court case: an MRI scan does not lie. It was clear to see where the injury had taken place. Unfortunately, I was not able to obtain a copy of his MRI scan to show here as the records are too old.

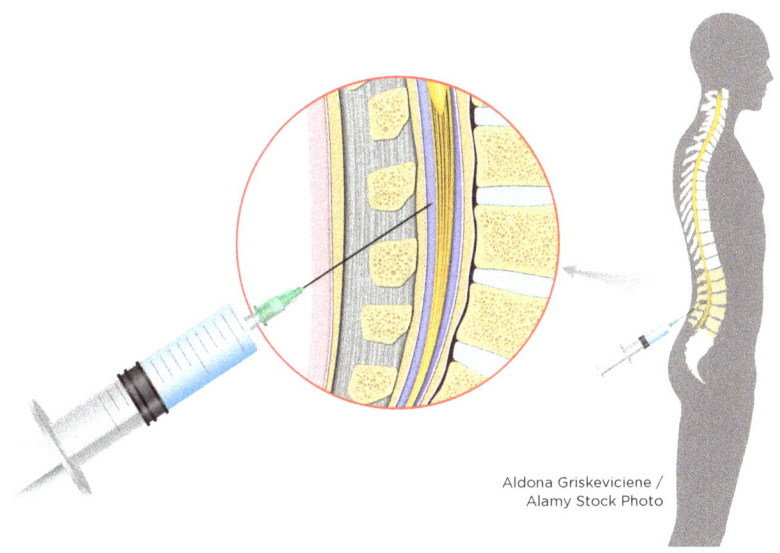

Aldona Griskeviciene / Alamy Stock Photo

Diagram 3. Lumbar puncture

A lumbar puncture (spinal tap) is a test used to diagnose certain health conditions. It is performed in the lower back, in the lumbar region. During a lumbar puncture, a needle is inserted into the space between two lumbar bones (vertebrae) to remove a sample of cerebrospinal fluid.

The procedure can help diagnose serious infections, disorders of the central nervous system, bleeding or cancers of the brain or spinal cord.

I don't really remember much more around this time. Perhaps the shock had finally kicked in and the trauma response over the years has taken some of these memories away. I know we had called our daughter who at this time was 15 years old and doing year 10 at high school. She caught the bus home, so there was one thing less for me to worry about with getting children home from school. I felt I was doing the right thing in not telling her too much. I didn't want her to have to worry about her dad. In hindsight, I probably should have been a lot more open with her. Perhaps that would have helped her to understand the pressures we were about to face.

It came as quite a shock that Peter had actually had a stroke. And we were then counting our blessings that he hadn't died and didn't appear to have any visually physical changes or disabilities, like a droopiness on one side of the face, or loss of feeling or movement down one side of the body. The long-term effects, however, would be another matter altogether.

Every day seemed to become a blur. We had so many questions – What had happened? Why had it happened? What do we do now? How will this affect us in the short and long term? These were issues which would have a huge impact on our everyday lives. Then the questions that arose: Will he be able to work again, and how will that affect our income? Will we have to sell our home? Will he be able to drive?

One thing that stood out for us was simply – it could have been a lot worse. A hell of a lot worse. So, keeping this in mind, we were optimistic that things would work out in the end. If only we had known just how long that would take.

It isn't until something like this happens that you start to think about all the smaller everyday details that may be adversely affected by an injury. If Peter had not been able to drive or even boil the kettle our lives would have been completely turned upside down as his care would have taken precedence over everything else. Having another close family friend suffer multiple strokes in recent years has certainly brought into sharp relief what a bullet we dodged and just how much lives can change because of the condition.

So back to the hospital – Peter was placed in the same ward where his father (less than 12 months earlier – December 2003) had passed away due to a stroke, so this added to the emotional trauma that we were all experiencing at that time. Thankfully he was not in the same room, but it was a little surprising that a couple of the nursing staff recognised Peter from his previous visits with his father.

A lot had been happening this year and I am not going to go into that side of the story as it has no bearing on what this book is about. One thing that still stands out today is a comment Peter said when I visited him one evening in hospital. He had this determined, and stern look on his face. I asked him what was wrong. His reply was simply that unless someone could bring something good and positive into our lives, they could take a very long walk off a very short plank (or words to that effect). We still hold to this sentiment today.

It was quite eye opening when we discovered how many people think the same way as we do in this regard. We came to realise which friends and family are valuable and those who were not. We had to cut some friends and family out of our lives for the sake of our mental health and wellbeing. It is something that should probably be reviewed every few years just to ensure that you are not gathering baggage. The same can be said to ensure that you maintain and nurture the people who have a positive influence in your life. They are the ones who will keep you going when the clouds descend.

CHAPTER 2

Picking up the pieces

After his hospital stay for a couple of weeks, Peter spent some time at home recovering and taking it easy. With the passing of his father in December 2003 and, not long after that, his grandmother (February 2004), then another short hospital stint for gall bladder problems (April 2004) before his stroke (August 2004), it was understandable that we really didn't want to do anything for the rest of the year. Peter especially had a lot to process, mentally and physically.

An important birthday, in more ways than one

Considering everything that had gone on and that he was just shy of his 40th birthday (early September) when he had the stroke, I decided to throw him a party regardless. We had to have something good and positive after everything else that had happened. I only invited people who we both decided brought those good and positive influences into our lives.

Dave and Jen were such friends who were, and still are, very important to us. At that time, they were living in Alice Springs. I didn't tell Peter that I had invited them. I let him think that they wouldn't be able to make it, which I was pretty sure was going to be the case, considering their work commitments and timing. On the morning of the party, I got a call from Jen to wish Peter an awesome day. I could hear their bird chirping away in the background, so I knew they were still at home in Alice Springs. My heart sank on realising they couldn't make it. Dave apparently had been called into work and wasn't available to speak to Peter but would call him later.

The party was going along very nicely, not too full on as Peter was still very tired and had to take it easy. Christine was running a little late as she had to duck back to work also to get some items (or so I was told). What we didn't know was Chris was in fact on her way to the airport to pick up Dave and Jen. They had done a major sneaky on us as a surprise for Peter. As Jen mentioned, Peter had been the best man at their wedding and there was no way they were not going to be there for him for his birthday, especially after everything that had happened.

It was the absolute highlight of Peter's week (and possibly his year really). We were both in tears to be seeing them as it was genuinely unexpected and everyone else was in on the secret except us. We certainly couldn't have asked for a stronger network of friends around us than those we kept and still have.

Permission to travel

By now Peter had been home from hospital for about 3 months and one thing that had become very apparent was how his body reacted to seasonal and weather changes. The change in air pressure just before a storm seemed to be the worst and was exhausting for him. We were coming into summer and the challenges were becoming obvious. Peter's mother Kathy thankfully convinced us that a holiday to the UK (during their winter) after all that happened that year was what we needed. So off we took late November 2004 for about 6 weeks to visit family in Chester and London. The cooler climate in those early days was just the trick. (Note: Peter had to get permission from his treating doctor to travel overseas. Because his stroke was injury-related and not hereditary/genetic, made this possible.

Seek advice from your own doctor before looking to travel.)

It must have been incredibly hard for Peter's mother (Kathy) at this time also as she had lost her husband less than a year earlier to a stroke (Robin passed away on their wedding anniversary of 47 years – 28 December 2003). Then Kathy's mother died on Valentine's Day, 2004. It was during the time of Great Grans funeral that Peter's Gall Bladder became septic and he wound up in hospital for an operation not long after. By the time our trip to England came around and looking back on all this now, I realise that my focus was completely on Peter and his health issues rather than the loss of Robin and Grandma and how Kathy may or may not be handling it all, considering her son also now (twice) in the same year had a close brush. It was not due to insensitivity, but simply trying to cope with the situation at the time. Peter was still alive, therefore he was the focus.

For me, again looking back on the time we were in England, it was probably the beginning of my own spiral into depression and anxiety. Having to 'keep it all together' for Kath, for our daughter, and for Peter, was certainly beginning to impact on me. The holiday itself had its ups and downs, I know I was on edge for most of the time away and Kathy was showing the first signs of dementia (though we didn't recognise it at the time, thinking it was most likely the stresses we had all been through that year, which in all fairness was probably a contributing factor). On the positive, the trip was just as much a healing process for us all as it was to spread my father-in-law's ashes at various places of deep meaning to them both.

I found myself requiring antidepressants (Zoloft) to help me get through. Having friends support is great, but they could not be with us 24/7, so reaching out and asking for help was a logical solution to an immediate problem. I remained on Zoloft until around 2016 when I gradually reduced and ceased my use of them. There have been times when I thought I should go back on them again, but another lesson we all learned over these past years is speaking up when things start to get challenging. Speaking about the difficulties I was experiencing has been therapeutic and I have not needed to go back to taking Zoloft.

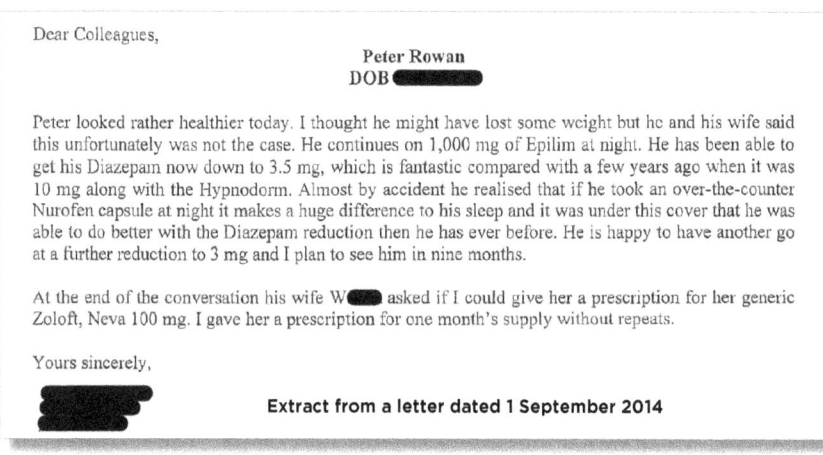

Dear Colleagues,

Peter Rowan
DOB ████

Peter looked rather healthier today. I thought he might have lost some weight but he and his wife said this unfortunately was not the case. He continues on 1,000 mg of Epilim at night. He has been able to get his Diazepam now down to 3.5 mg, which is fantastic compared with a few years ago when it was 10 mg along with the Hypnodorm. Almost by accident he realised that if he took an over-the-counter Nurofen capsule at night it makes a huge difference to his sleep and it was under this cover that he was able to do better with the Diazepam reduction then he has ever before. He is happy to have another go at a further reduction to 3 mg and I plan to see him in nine months.

At the end of the conversation his wife W███ asked if I could give her a prescription for her generic Zoloft, Neva 100 mg. I gave her a prescription for one month's supply without repeats.

Yours sincerely,

Extract from a letter dated 1 September 2014

A work opportunity

I happened to bump into Neil just before we went away. Peter had worked for Neil previously for several years, so naturally he asked after us all. I gave him a run-down of our crappy year and told him we were about to head over to the UK to get away for a while. Neil asked me to get Peter to call him when we got back as he may be able to help out with some work.

Upon our return, we reached out to him, and he was able to offer Peter a contract job with himself as his boss again.

Knowing Peter's current condition, Neil was able to assist him in navigating his retained and lost knowledge. He worked for Neil for a few years between early 2005 to around mid 2008.

I recall Peter telling me about a particular day at work where one of the other IT consultants asked a question about some specific program. Peter immediately responded with the information required to complete the task. The moment he said it, there was silence from Neil and their associate and shocked looks on their faces. Neil asked Peter, 'Where did that come from?' Peter was just as shocked as they were. It was information that he didn't think he would know or remember considering his injury. It highlighted once again just how much random information was still in there and clearly there were pathways damaged, some not and some perhaps finding a different route to information needed.

It was good for Peter also to have a purpose again. Sadly, he was not able to retain long-term employment in his condition, especially when Neil moved on from his role. His brain injury left so many disconnections that a lot of information vital to his role was simply lost as the pathways for them were gone. We will of course be forever grateful to Neil for the time Peter was able to work as it allowed us some financial relief as well as the time to navigate the presenting symptoms and finding ways to manage them accordingly.

Peter had, over the years, looked at going back to some form of paid work, but the challenges with his recovery really made him unreliable with attendance, so it was basically put on the back-burner. Due to the brain injury, it became pretty obvious that he could no longer quantify his years of experience in the

IT industry and he would never return to that again. There were just too many gaps in his knowledge.

Sometime around 2010, a friend of Peter's introduced him to another friend of hers who was struggling to keep up with some of the demands within his own business. As this was around electronics and cabling, it was potentially something Peter could assist him with – being bulk and repetitive work. A meeting was set up with Howard to discuss what he did and how Peter may be able to relieve some of the load for him. The work was very intermittent and repetitive. This was fine for Peter as he effectively didn't really have to think too much about a constantly changing platform, and he could do the work at his own pace from home. It was a win–win situation for everyone as it freed up a lot of Howard's time, allowing him to concentrate on sourcing more business. The work is still coming in all these years later, but it remains very intermittent. We consider it pocket money for Peter now and it gives him something to do outside of the household activities.

CHAPTER 3

Presenting symptoms: Memory, Fatigue, Anger and Depression

Memory

Peter noticed he was struggling to remember some words. He could picture what he wanted to say but couldn't remember how to formulate the sentence. It came down to basic training again as you would with a child. Stop, take a deep breath, think about what you want to say first, then verbalise. I can't remember how long it took for him to reconnect that part of his memory, I do know it was gradual, but certainly not the most pressing issue he had so we didn't really focus a lot on it.

The memory loss initially occurred at the same time as the damage to various parts of his brain. It just took time to understand exactly which parts of his memory were missing. Usually, it involved us talking about a particular time, place or event for him (and us) to realise he couldn't recall what had transpired at that time. It simply took time and repetition to get back to mostly normal again, though when it comes to some things like events that happened some time ago, he is better off looking at photos to jog his memory into recall.

Other everyday little things were presenting as a struggle – putting the car keys down somewhere or his glasses, or a mug, for example. He may have only just put it in the 'usual spot' but couldn't remember actually putting the item there. He describes it now as having brain fog. It's easy to say this is a common thing with everyone, but it is also really important to understand how the stroke may damage areas of the brain. In Peter's case there were still connections, but some of them had become dead ends. There were some totally random things he would remember and others that completely escaped him that he should have known. It's like having to travel across the country without a map. You know what direction you need to go, but which road do you take that doesn't lead you to a dead end or turn you around. The frustration levels would fluctuate during this time and I am sure he beat himself up a bit over it. He did often comment, 'I should know this stuff!' and the frustration was evident in his voice.

Of course, it was always painful to remind him of the fact that he'd had a brain injury and it was going to take time. In this, Peter was not very patient. He seemed to retain his logical and critical thinking and his mechanical ability but struggled with dates and events (like attending weddings, birthdays and holidays). The disconnections in his brain were very random. We did take a lot of photos when travelling in England (and Japan on the final leg coming home), which was very useful for his memory. Seeing the pictures helped trigger some memories for him, though not all of them. He just accepted that if he was in the photo, he must have been there.

I am grateful though that he remembered how to boil the kettle and cook.

Once Peter left work permanently (around 4 years after his stroke), and while I was still leaving the house to go to work, his memory was presenting a bit more as a problem. Peter was always well domesticated and helpful around the house, but he was at a point where he just didn't register that something needed to be done before I got home – taking something out of the freezer for dinner for example. Although I may have asked him to do something before I left, he simply forgot. It didn't even register to him that I *had* asked him to do something. Again, it is important to remember that when a stroke happens – and it can be different for everyone – there will be some brain damage. What gets damaged can vary greatly. The only way we could combat this was to simply write a list every day of anything I wanted him to do – washing, ironing, vacuuming, and so on. Sometimes everything was done, sometimes it wasn't. Which was perfectly fine as we were also navigating how much he could push himself each day. It was very frustrating for him that he couldn't do everything he used to do before. (I address this more when discussing 'Navigating the depression and anger' on p. 31). So this now leads to fatigue.

Fatigue

Doing basic housework gave Peter a purpose every day. He really only had two choices at this time. Sit and dwell on what happened or find something to distract him. Doing housework solved two problems for us – it gave him something to do and helped me out considering I was out for most of the day.

The challenges to his body due to the change in weather continued to be a problem and there was no way I could expect anything to get done around the house on those days. We mentioned these seasonal difficulties to his neurologist who had heard of this from a few of his patients and he said he would probably have to do a study on this phenomenon.

Peter still tried to push himself to do more, but when the result came with 3 to 4 days of being so tired and weak that he slept for most of the day, he finally stopped trying to 'man up' and started to take an active role in getting himself back on track. And if this meant doing only what I told him to do and nothing more, so be it. It was also very important for him to listen to his own body and recognise if he couldn't do anything on a particular day. The communication between us at this time started to improve greatly. He listened to me when I told him no (to doing anything too physical – like mowing the lawn), and he let me know when he felt he just shouldn't do anything for a day or two. On those days he tended to stay inside in the air conditioning, perhaps watching TV, reading or sleeping. Any form of housework he did (if at all) was all very light and low priority.

The in-between times over the early years and after he ceased working full time (from 2008), he spent some time with a friend at Kellyville church doing craft days. A very dear friend of mine was teaching lead-lighting and Peter had an interest in this, so he attended the lessons whenever he could. This was good for him on many levels – besides getting him out of the house on those days, he had some social time and had a focus on something that he had to concentrate on. With what he learned during the classes he brought home and spent some time a few years later (after we had moved in 2012) making a couple of panels to go into our front door. Sadly, I'm still waiting for them to be fitted, but perfection takes time and if anything, we have learned to be patient.

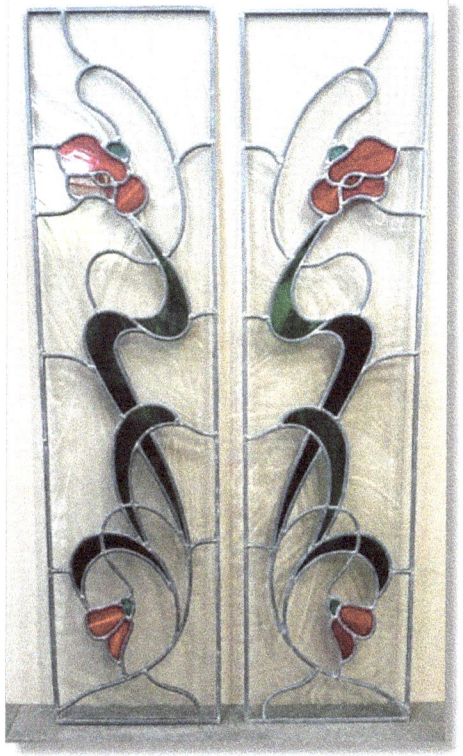

Peter made a matching pair of these panels and I hope to one day see them fitted to our front door.

Medications and their side effects

Peter's medication really became a focal point during his fatigue. These are the drugs he was prescribed:
- Hypnodorm (flunitrazepam): used to treat severe cases of insomnia
- Ducene (diazepam): treatment for short-term anxiety, helps relax nerves cells and calms the brain)
- Valium (also a type of diazepam with similar effects): to help with sleep initially. This had to be boosted with Epilim

- Epilim (sodium valproate): generally used for the treatment of epilepsy but may also be used to control mania, a mental condition with episodes of overactivity, elation or irritability. Peter needed it to slow his brain activity down after it was found he was processing the Hypnodorm within a very short time frame (12 hours) and there appeared to be no additional relief in the following hours.

You would think that a brain injury would already slow his brain activity down, but unfortunately for him, it had the opposite effect. It appeared that other parts of his brain were compensating for the damaged areas and things ramped up (a tinnitus-type sound – I address this on p. 34). This was a real issue at night when everything else was quiet. The medication became a blessing and a curse to some degree. He was only meant to be on the diazepam for a maximum of 4 months, but it took us several years to wean him off this.

Looking back again to our time in the UK during winter and as mentioned above, his fatigue appeared to be seasonal; we found we could really only change his medication effectively and reduce the use of the addictive diazepam during the winter months.

There were more side effects that presented themselves, which we now believe were due to the combination of medications he was taking. Peter was never formally diagnosed with Irritable Bowel Syndrome or Coeliac disease, but one afternoon when speaking to a girlfriend about her symptoms of being a Coeliac, there were too many similarities with Peter's symptoms, so we wondered if he was suffering that also. Rather than going to a doctor to be diagnosed, Peter decided to cut gluten from his diet altogether – just initially as a trial run. This wasn't a terribly hard task as we ate a lot of fruit, veg and fresh meat as it was. We substituted bread and pasta with the gluten free varieties. Once we started looking it was easy enough to find gluten free options to most of what we ate anyway and what we couldn't find, or simply found too expensive, we just cut out. Over time things were tweaked and we found that some gluten products didn't seem to affect him – gravy was one that comes to mind.

The other side effect was little fluid blisters that appeared on his hands, mostly on the palm and in the creases. They were incredibly itchy and at the height of irritation actually split his skin. There were some mornings he would wake unable to open his hand due to a formed scab on the wound. We visited many skin specialists and tried everything under the sun including herbal remedies. Nothing worked and he began to accept that this was just another thing he would have to live with. Thankfully it was only a few years in the scheme of it all and once his medication was lessening, so was the irritation. Like the stomach aches he got from eating gluten, perhaps this skin irritation was also a by-product of the medication mix.

On a side note, we were walking past a bakery one day (this was about 10 to 12 years after the incident) and Peter commented that he was really craving a good old meat pie. He hadn't had one in years since he gave up gluten. I told him to get one as we were not away anywhere on the weekend and if he wound up in the bathroom all weekend so what. The least he should do is enjoy every single mouthful. As it was, he ate the pie, didn't sit in the bathroom all weekend and didn't have any cramps! As we did with everything that happened to his body over the years, we started to analyse why this may be so and the only thing we could pinpoint it to was the reduction and in some cases the elimination of the medication. We didn't want to push this lightbulb moment, so he waited another couple of weeks before trying a pie again. Same thing. All good. We didn't want to shock his system with a flood of gluten products again, so bit by bit we slowly introduced things back into his diet again and as of today he is completely free to eat whatever he wants again. This is only a small win, but a win nonetheless and a reminder to never stop trying and never give up hope even on the little things.

The only other thing that has been affected by Peter's fatigue is of course our sex life. Whenever things did get intimate, it wore him out so much, that afterwards he was just too tired for anything else. Needless to say, intimacy at that level reduced quite significantly. It's a good thing we can both enjoy each other's company, and this didn't break our relationship. I know that this part of our lives played on Peter's mind and probably at times made him feel 'less of a man'. Accepting that this was a current reality and not necessarily a forever adjustment is really the only way you can manage something like this. With so many other things that were affecting him at various levels, at least this was something we could manage to help reduce his fatigue so we could focus on healing other areas of his injury.

Looking back, the first 7 to 9 years were probably the worst for Peter simply because he had been so active in so many areas of his life, and after the stroke he found himself struggling with everyday simple tasks. I have to admit that I found this frustrating also. The sudden pressures to keep everything moving, bills paid, mortgage paid, sanity in check as other aspects of our life didn't stop just because Peter had a stroke. At times it was overwhelming, and this is where having close

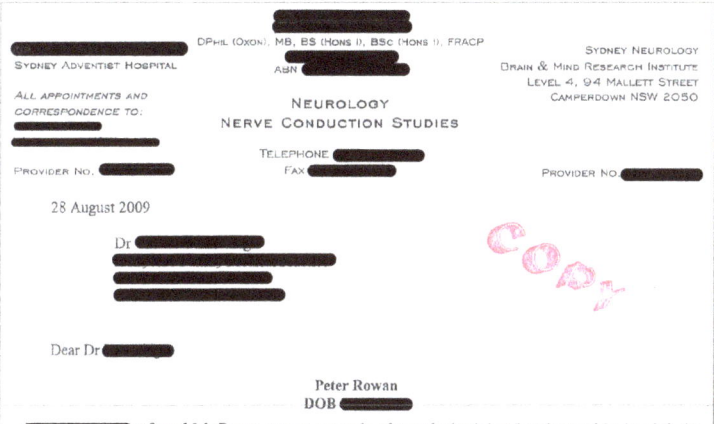

NEUROLOGY
NERVE CONDUCTION STUDIES

28 August 2009

Dear Dr

Peter Rowan
DOB

referred Mr Rowan to me a couple of months back but I understand he has left the practice. Mr Rowan came along today with his wife. I had previously seen him for medicolegal reasons. His court case was settled back in March - he wanted to see me now as a treating doctor and I was happy to do so in his case. The principal problems are fatigue and insomnia. He takes 2 mg of Hypnodorm at night, 10 mg of Diazepam at night, 400 mg of Epilim at night and 5 mg of Visken at night. The Visken has been prescribed for about two years, originally 5 mg twice a day but his blood pressure has been reasonably good lately.

He has given up work entirely.

Today he looked well, perhaps a little downcast. The blood pressure was 108/70 mmHg in the right arm.

Visken like all the betablockers is known for causing sleep disturbance, insomnia, vivid dreams etc and I think the first move should be to stop the Visken immediately. He may not need an antihypertensive but to be sure in his case given his history would you be able to arrange a 24 hour blood pressure measurement in a couple of weeks so we can get a "real world" idea what his blood pressure is like?

If he needs to be on a medication I would prescribe it from one of the other classes.

The next move that I have suggested is to increase the Epilim by one tablet, to 600 mg at night. This may benefit his mood, and could add a little to night time sedation. After this I plan to see him in about six weeks, hoping to start weaning his benzodiazepines. If this plan goes well most of it could take place under your direction.

2

Depending on how these manoeuvres end up he may also do well with a small dose of the tricyclic antidepressant Amitriptyline. He has been on a number of antidepressants over the years but none from this class as far as he can remember. Sometimes 10 to 25 mg of Amitriptyline is all that people need to get to sleep better and stay asleep; this effect appears not to wear off, contrary to the benzodiazepines.

I think I can make a difference but I have warned him that it will take a few months.

Yours sincerely,

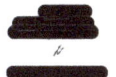

Extracts from neurologist correspondence to supervising GP, 28 August 2009

friends to call on really did save our lives on many levels.

Fatigue, anger and depression all started to meld during this time and was becoming quite toxic to Peter's mental wellbeing. It was about 4 years into his condition that we sought legal help (2007 to 2008). It took about 3 years for all the symptoms to present themselves and we really began to understand just how much damage had been done and the lifelong ripple effect this was possibly going to cause: His insomnia, lack of energy, itchy hands, memory loss, problems with his diet. As mentioned earlier though, I am not going to go into the legal details. The anger Peter felt at what had happened, not just towards the chiropractor who caused the injury, but at himself for his current situation began to compound and this is where his depression started to take hold.

Peter has since commented that the first 10 years were probably his most frustrating.

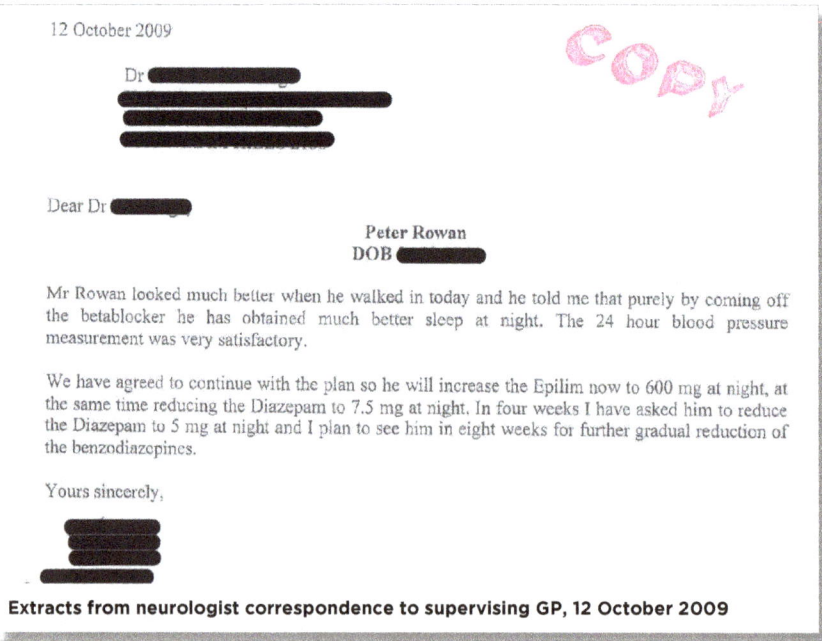

Extracts from neurologist correspondence to supervising GP, 12 October 2009

Navigating the depression and anger

Life is about choices. Some we regret, some we're proud of. We are what we choose to be.

GRAHAM BROWN

Peter was brought up in the typical 1960s Australian way, meaning he didn't complain, he 'sucked it up', he 'faced it like a man', kept a 'stiff upper lip' and any other idiom you can think of. Because of this he tended to suffer in silence. The type of man he is meant he also didn't want me to worry about him and the frustrations he was facing every day. It took quite a while for Peter to finally let go of holding everything in and express how he was feeling each day. The path to get to this was quite rocky at times and for a man who tended towards silence, he would express his frustration by getting quite impatient at some things. He never lashed out physically, but you could see in his whole state that he was wound up. He would always go off somewhere quietly when it got too much, which in itself could exacerbate the sound in his head. This then usually resulted in the kettle being put on, along with some music (playing a little louder than usual), probably in an attempt to drown out the sound in his head.

We found also that once we started to make more proactive tweaks with his medication, his sleep improved a bit. That had an overall positive ripple effect with his mood and overall outlook – if one area could show signs of improvement, then there are chances so could other areas. It just took an incredibly long time to find the balance and it seemed that the goal posts were constantly changing. Sometimes it was two steps forward and one step back. As mentioned earlier, it was mostly during winter where we could have a positive impact with changes in his medication. Sometimes during summer, it went back again and we had to endure another year before we could perhaps take another step forward.

> Mr Rowan is going well. He came along today with his wife. He found 600 mg of Epilim a night a little too much and was able to drop to 500 mg – I gave him a prescription for this. He has now managed to halve his Ducene to 5 mg at night and I have asked him to reduce this further over the next month, by a half tablet initially. If he finds the drop too much I am happy for him to go for a more gradual reduction.
>
> Assuming the Ducene cessation goes as planned, in early February I want to start reducing the Hypnodorm. He currently takes two of the 1 mg tablets in the evening. I have asked him to reduce this by a quarter tablet, with review here in March.
>
> **Extract from neurologist correspondence to supervising GP: 7 December 2009**

> He had trouble staying on a lower dose of Ducene and had to go back up to 5 mg at night but he is going to start reducing it again tonight. However he has had more luck in reducing the Hypnodorm from 2 mg regularly to 1.5 mg. The reduction will have to be slow and I expect there may be the occasional set back.
>
> He is still on 500 mg of Epilim at night, not being able to tolerate 600 mg before but I think as the benzodiazepines come down he may need more Epilim e.g 600-700 mg and in fact he may be able to tolerate more Epilim so it is going to be quite a tricky job finessing this situation, but I think we can do it.
>
> I would like to see him again in three months.
>
> **Extract from neurologist correspondence to supervising GP: 12 March 2010**

The things that helped

Thankfully Peter wasn't opposed to doing the housework, cooking, cleaning, washing and ironing. Apart from removing the burden from me, the really good thing that came out of this was his appreciation for working parents whose partners didn't contribute to keeping house, especially when children were involved. I believe it was this realisation that was just one turning point that started to bring him back from the edge. It also gave him a reason to keep going each day, even when, on some of those days, he was just a breath away from going over that edge. He once commented to me about one of our friends who at the time was a single mum with three schoolboys, working full time and fitting in sporting activities, wondering how she managed on her own.

I think it was an eye opener for him to understand that although he was not working to earn money and contributing to the household financially, he was certainly contributing to our everyday lives in very significant ways, even if it is hard to put a monetary figure on keeping the home together. Once he understood just how much he did contribute – and this increased quite significantly once the realisation was there on how much time it took to keep house – we were able to start focusing once again on continuing his improvements.

The things that didn't help

Working on the garden, however, was the one thing he could not attend to regularly, especially during summer. It simply drained him too much, as the humidity and change in air pressure made him incredibly tired, and when there was a thunderstorm brewing on the horizon, it was all the worse.

Then came the realisation for both of us, that Peter would not be able to return to work, especially in the role he was gainfully employed for previously. Trying to find other work was a struggle simply because we never knew when he was going to have an 'off' day. It was a major knock to his self-esteem. His fatigue and depression played a large part in this. I think he felt a bit of guilt that I had to work to look after him. Being a little 'old school', he felt that he should be able to get better and go back to work. I'm sure it was quite a shock to him when the realisation hit home that that was never going to happen.

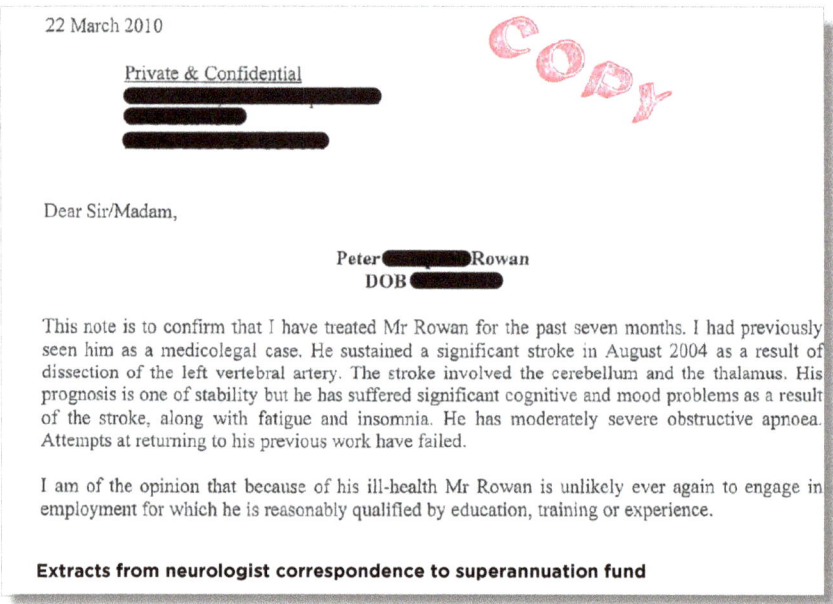

Extracts from neurologist correspondence to superannuation fund

Tinnitus

Besides the (undiagnosed) gluten intolerance which we were managing and his ability to understand the weather conditions and adjust his daily energy expenditure accordingly, the biggest issue he had then and still has to this day is an 'audio generated sound' in his head. I'll say tinnitus as this is a common ailment that most people can understand. Tinnitus, however, is usually located in the ears and is caused by broken or damaged hair cells in the part of the ear that receives sound (the cochlea). There are other factors that can cause tinnitus, but for this purpose, I'll only mention this one. In Peter's case, he had hearing tests done and all came back normal, his 'tinnitus' appeared to be caused by the damage done to his thalamus. This one thing alone has been a constant irritation to a point that at one time he became suicidal.

Most people have some form of tinnitus, and it can be at varying degrees of intensity and can switch on and off at any given time. Imagine having cicadas buzzing in your head at the height of their season 24 hours a day, 7 days a week and 365 days a year. It would be enough to drive anyone out of their mind.

This was another hurdle to overcome and try to 'fix'. Sorry to say, it has never been fixed and to this day is still an ongoing problem. There was only one day in the past 19 years that I can recall when Peter told me that the noises had stopped in one ear only. That time he happened to have a bit of a head cold. The look of amazement on his face was incredible and we hoped beyond hope that the noise would stay switched off. It didn't last long, but perhaps that is something to ponder further. I just don't really like the idea of forcing another head cold to find out.

We had to do something. Peter tried hypnotherapy which did help, but the ongoing cost of treatment just couldn't be maintained. The only other option we came up with was 'white noise'. Thankfully the iPod was fairly new on the market and seemed like a good option to try. It appeared to work only to a point of offering relief. The most beneficial time was at night when he was trying to get to sleep. When everything was quiet at night, the noise in his ears would 'ramp up' and contributed to his inability to sleep despite the medication he was on. It took him a while, but after trolling through many genres of music, he found that Dance and Techno styles had the best effect for him. This style was the complete opposite to what he usually listened to and preferred, but who was to complain if it provided the desired effect – relief.

Although wearing iPod earbuds at night was very beneficial for him, he found wearing them during the day and when at functions also helped. It enabled him to focus on people talking to him as the noise in his head was subdued, especially if it was a large gathering like a birthday or wedding. The background noise from many voices in an enclosed area on top of the constant buzzing in his head made it very hard to concentrate and focus on a conversation. If the crowds were too noisy then the buzzing in his ears was very prominent for at least a few days after the event. The iPod helped in limiting the amount of 'clutter' that got in and therefore lowered the chance of him having intense buzzing for further days ahead. By having the iPod earbuds in, his brain was subconsciously focusing on the music rather than external noises (clutter) and gave him the opportunity to focus on the conversations and stop his brain from being overwhelmed.

Of course, this also raised another set of complications – people's response to him using an iPod, especially at a wedding, for example. We would often see people looking at him in disgust or anger that 'he had the audacity to be listening to music when there was an important speech happening'. It became quite draining having to tell people why he was using an iPod and that he was not being rude. Then the looks of disdain turned to pity which was almost as bad. As a result, Peter didn't want to go out so often, because he didn't want to have to constantly explain himself and verbalise the frustration he was going through. Talking about his current issues with people just brought back into focus his struggles. If he was at a wedding, he wanted to be able to relax and (with the help of the iPod) have an opportunity to not hear or drown out a bit of the constant buzz. When he had to explain himself (or for the most part, I explained for him), it was a reminder that the sound was there and he had to start again to try and push the sound away so he could enjoy himself for a short moment. He started going out less and less which gave him a feeling of isolation, and this just added to his unstable state of mind.

Dizziness/Balance

Peter found that every time he went to bed or closed his eyes in the first 12–18 months he felt the sensation of 'bed spins'. No matter where he was, whenever he shut his eyes he felt a sensation of falling backwards and to his left. This was an issue every time he had a shower when rinsing shampoo out of his hair for example. The only way he could combat that in this situation was to lean against the wall or place his hand on the wall as a point of reference – giving his brain something to focus on as a grounding point. For the first 6–12 months Peter rarely drove purely from a safety aspect, and if he did, he was not alone in the vehicle. Once he was able to adjust himself to this sensation and felt confident in driving again, he would do very short trips to the local shops and progressively built up his confidence and distance of travel. So long as his eyes were open and he had points of reference he was ok. The medication over the years helped with him being able to mentally and physically adjust to these sensations and over time the severity has reduced. Thankfully Peter was able to adapt to these sensations otherwise he would not have been able to work for Neil or confidently drive again. Looking back on this area of his condition and subsequent improvement again is a reminder that when an injury is suffered, healing will take time and you should always be mindful of your limitations. Don't take unnecessary risks during the healing process.

The darkest times

His depression due to the sound in his head was really taking its toll. Even now on really bad days it still brings him down. On one particularly bad morning, he told me he was ready to swallow the whole lot (of his medication) just to put an end to it (around 2008 to 2009). This was a real wake-up call to me that showed just how much everything was building up for him. As mentioned earlier, Peter kept a lot to himself probably to shelter me from having worry about him so much, but the tinnitus sound was more than he could handle on top of everything else. I immediately told his doctor, the chemist and our neurologist what he had said. The chemist was under strict direction to not hand any medication to him and only provide it to me, his mother or our daughter for safe keeping. It was also during this time that, after discussion with the neurologist, we set a path to specifically wean him off everything, not just the diazepam. Remember, it took 7 years to get him off the diazepam that he should have only been on for a few months.

I started paying a lot more attention to how Peter was looking and feeling from day to day and his reactions to what was happening as a general everyday including weather changes. It was hard to determine if the noise in his head ramped up more under any specific conditions. It appeared to be quite random, but when he was suitably distracted it seemed to lessen a little. Not so much as going away as not being in the forefront and focused on. The days that he appeared to be at his worst were the days I called on our dear friend Dave.

CHAPTER 4

Friendships

Love is our true destiny. We do not find the meaning of life by ourselves alone. We find it with another.

THOMAS MERTON

Dave and Peter had met in 1996 when attending TAFE to get their private pilot licences. Something just clicked with them and they have been firm friends ever since. We found out some years later that his partner's (now wife's) family were also friends with some members of my own family, so it really was only a matter of time before ships passing in the night met up. It was Dave's sister-in-law Christine who I called upon on the fateful day to meet me at the hospital.

Sadly, Peter had to give away his love for flying. The tinnitus sound in his head made it challenging to hear instructions or calls on the radio and purely from a safety aspect, he stopped flying. He was out one day with his instructor (although by this time he was licenced to fly solo) and there was an instruction sent through their radio which he did not respond to or acknowledge. His instructor asked him if he heard what was said, to which he replied he had not. That was the crunch for him to give up flying. It was a real shame as this was one thing he really enjoyed, but safety at all levels was certainly far more important.

Dave, his wife Jen and both their families really became the mainstay in helping Peter get out of the house and start living again. They all knew exactly what Peter was going through and (not ignoring it) didn't constantly remind him of this fact. Peter could 'be himself' without having to explain. On Peter's worst days when Dave was available and I asked him to come over, there were no assumptions, it was just purely a distraction to calm the storm that was beginning to boil. The visit may have included pottering around the garden, tinkering on a car, watching a movie, reading a car magazine, any number of things. It is the quiet support that seemed to just ease the tension, let you breathe so once again you can function. As I've said before, I simply don't know where we would be today if it wasn't for this support from genuine friends. There are very few people in the world who can honestly say that they trust someone (I'm talking about friends and family) with their lives.

Friendship isn't about who you have known the longest, it's about those who came and never left your side.
UNKNOWN

You will find that when something dramatic happens in your life, your true friends/family will really shine through, and you will find support in some of the most unexpected places. Restating what Peter said when I visited him in hospital: 'Unless someone can bring something good and positive into our lives, they can take a long walk'. Don't be sad if you have to cut people out of your life in these circumstances, and don't apologise for focusing on your own health – mental and/or physical. If those people are to remain in your life they will come back, but not before you are ready. We had to cut out some people who had been family friends for 40 years and even my father, which may horrify some people. I'm only mentioning this so you know it is ok. I have no regrets and these decisions enabled us to positively focus on the most important element in our lives and that was Peter's recovery. We just didn't need the negative impacts from other areas.

A couple of years after Peter had his stroke, he decided to get a tattoo to commemorate the important things in our lives – specifically the immediate family unit – him, me and our daughter. Our daughter and I both got the same tattoo as well. This is a permanent reminder that no matter what struggles we go through in life, there are people who will always be by our side no matter what. One long-term family 'friend' saw the tattoo on our daughter and immediately took offence and walked out of our home. It didn't matter to her that it represented something a lot deeper than a simple inking. Yes, that person was also cut out of our lives. As I said earlier, when something dramatic happens in your life, your true rocks will reveal themselves.

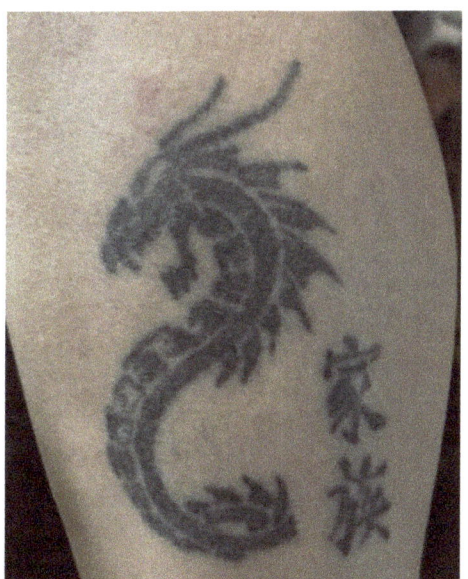

Kazoku
Translated means 'Family'.

CHAPTER 5

Moving forward some more

September 2009, I found myself changing careers again to enable me to work more from home. The main reason for this total change in career for me was because my previous job took me away from home for a week at a time on a very regular basis – home for a week, away for a week, home for another week and away again. One morning whilst travelling through the northern area of the territory that I managed, a vehicle was travelling toward me on my side of the road. It was a very close call and shook me terribly. Two more times on that same trip I had close encounters. It was the catalyst for me to get off the road, away from travel and take control of how often and when I was away from home. I was working in this role from around mid-2006 to December 2008. I did take some time off to spend with Peter before starting my new role around August/September 2009.

This was around the time that Peter opened up about wanting take all of his tablets at once just to make it all stop. Starting up one's own business is a stress in itself and led us to having to sell our family home a couple of years later in 2011. We did buy another property that was slightly less than what we had sold for, so we had a buffer whilst I was still growing my own business – 14 years later and I am still going so that is a good thing.

This was the first time we had bought an already-established home so there were a few things that needed fixing up on it. It is an older home on a large suburban block which was good for the dogs and something new for Peter to spend some focus on. As mentioned previously, he hadn't lost his ability to think logically or mechanically and he had always been quite good at building and renovating, so the challenge of this property was probably good timing. It was with this property over the coming years that Peter was really able to start on his fatigue and build up his fitness levels again.

The 15-year mark

It has taken me 15 years for my body to adjust and stabilise to the point that I can manage my energy levels again and I can recognise the symptoms of fatigue and depression and when I need to take time out.

PETER

At around the 15-year mark from Peter's initial injury, we visited with his neurologist again for the last time. He was really happy with Peter's progress and to some degree surpassed expectations on his recovery. Hearing him tell Peter there is no longer a need for him to keep seeing him was a momentous moment for Peter. He wasn't 100 percent recovered, and probably never will be, but recovered as much as he was going to be at that point in time and anything more was really now up to us. By this time, Peter had been completely weaned off the medication including the Epilim, Ducene and the Valium for around 12 months. (Peter had been on medication for around

14 years! Changes will not happen overnight. It is going to take a long time and one step at a time.) In the summertime we watched for changes in air pressure from impending storms and on those days, he spent inside in the air conditioning with the dogs, a movie or listening to music.

> **Peter Rowan**
> **DOB** ▉▉▉▉▉
>
> As I said last year Peter looked quite marvellous. He confirmed that he is going well.
>
> He has been off the Valium for over a year and was off the Epilim for a long time before that too so he is taking no regular medications. He is looking after his diet. He has lost about 6 kg of weight and is physically very active with renovations and currently building some pretty significant garden beds for vegetables. He has an occasional headache, perhaps no more than once every six weeks and still finds Nurofen can help. He has not needed to try Imigran. I am very happy with his progress - this has been an excellent outcome for a rather long journey.
>
> We do not think he needs regular review but I will fit him in at short notice should something come up.
>
> Yours sincerely,
>
> **Extracts from neurologist correspondence to supervising GP, 12 October 2019**

Our home, which we have been in now for coming up to 12 years, is still a work in progress, and probably will be for another century the way we are going, but there is no rush and we have always done things here at Peter's pace which has allowed him to slowly build up his stamina over time.

The SES

A couple of years after our last visit with the neurologist, Peter decided he needed to do something more rather than being stuck at home with me and the dogs all the time. Clearly, he would never be going back to paid work and certainly not in the IT industry where he had worked previously. Doing the intermittent work for Howard satisfied him to a degree and at least gave him meaning and purpose. Our circle of friends remained tight, but they also had lives to lead and, in some cases, moved further away from the family nest, including our daughter, so social interaction was on the decline for him. The challenge was finding something that would hold his interest for the long term, didn't cost a fortune as a new 'hobby' might, and allowed him to get out of the house on occasion. So, he joined the local SES around October 2019. It was a win–win situation. It meant he was taking himself out of his current comfort zone, forcing himself to meet other people and giving something back to the local community. Being a volunteer also meant he could pace himself on how involved he wanted to be. Almost 4 years later and he is still involved and has met some really lovely people along the way.

COVID of course interfered with some of his training, which took a few years to complete instead of the usual 6 to 12 months. Thankfully Peter's stroke didn't upset his usual level of patience. Since being with SES he has trained for on-water flood rescue, urban search and rescue, industrial and domestic rescue, road crash rescue, large animal and general land rescue. His current training includes vertical rescue. It would be fair to say he has become an integral part of the team. He has obtained one stripe for his rescue activities and is on his way to earning his second. He is now officially recognised with the State Rescue Board as a general land rescue operator. Certainly, something I am very proud of and so is he.

What now?

There are always going to be some residual issues, the biggest one for Peter still being the audio generated sound in his head, but having lived with everything else for so long, you eventually begin to subconsciously adjust as required. The important thing he does here is not stop whilst he can keep going, whether this be as a local volunteer, getting more renovations done that I can dream up on the way, or anything to keep his mind and body active. There are days when the sound in his head is torture and he struggles. On those days the distractions are required even more, so I'm glad there are still renovations to be done to keep him distracted; along with the fact that we are on a fairly large block that requires constant maintenance.

It took Peter over 15 years to get back some semblance of a normal life. An injury like this does not heal overnight, in 6 months or even a year. There are so many adjustments that need to be made on a physical, mental and emotional level that at times can be incredibly overwhelming. It was important for us to remember 'it could have been a lot worse'. The fact that he can drive, wash, walk, even talk without any noticeable impairments is a bonus on many levels.

Dealing with criticism, disbelief and doubts about his mental and physical stability was very challenging at times and still can be on occasion. Someone may look perfectly fine but be a total mess inside. I was asked once what type of chocolate Peter would be – I said a Flake – looks all smooth and normal on the outside while it is all over the place on the inside.

The challenges are still ongoing, but at least now, 19 years later it is not all-consuming. We have finally found a relatively happy balance in our lives and continue to enjoy every day he is still with us.

Peter mentioned to me recently that he has found a great sense of achievement with obtaining his first stripe for rescue with SES and looking forward to adding another stripe sometime in the near future. He is so proud of everything he has achieved since getting the all-clear from the neurologist and giving back to the community in a voluntary way is very rewarding mentally and physically for him.

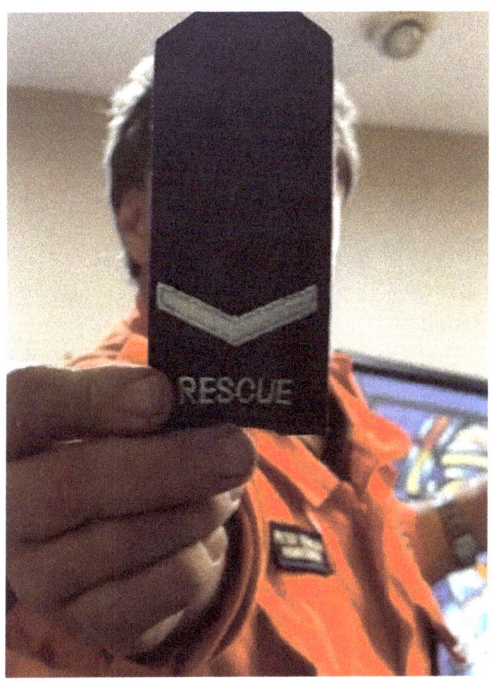

I feel a new purpose with what I do with the SES team. I can't go back to work for many reasons and certainly not in the field I was originally doing. Being a volunteer gives me the flexibility I need to help me manage my health, but also the drive to get up and get out and do something constructive and worthwhile.

PETER

CHAPTER 6

Things I have learned

Do you have a will?

It is really important to point out that neither of us had a will at the time of Peter's stroke and if the worst had happened, who knew what level of financial strife we would have been in. Quite commonly people will say 'Oh, I don't have enough assets to get one of them'. But that is not true. Anyone who is working, whether still living at home or not, will have superannuation, possibly some furniture, a vehicle, savings, and so on. You do have assets.

The same can be said for have an Enduring Power of Attorney (EPOA). If you haven't implemented either of these items, talk to a solicitor now so you understand the difference between a POA (Power of Attorney) and an EPOA.

A POA or EPOA are just as important, if not more so, than a will – your life is your biggest asset.

Both Peter and I have these in place now and the relief you get from knowing it is done cannot be measured.

Do you have life insurance?

One of the last things people consider, and usually the first to be cut due to budgeting, is life insurance.

People insure their cars and their homes as 'they are the most expensive assets we own'. I think it would be fair to say that our lives and our ability to earn income are far more valuable assets. Some people never think about, or sadly care, what sort of financial and mental state they will leave themselves and their loved ones in if the worst were to happen, and it's not usually until we are faced with our own mortality that we stop to look at what did happen or could have happened and what we need to get done and should have had in place already.

If you suffer and survive a trauma and you have no insurance at all, you will quickly start to care. Quite often an insurance company won't cover you for some medical conditions or traumas if they are pre-existing. So the horse has bolted and it's now too late.

Take some time to review what you have, discuss with a professional advisor (financial planner/advisor or an accredited insurance provider) about what you may/may not need and remember, *some insurance is better than none.*

Afterword

The years have been challenging on many levels and this really is only a snippet of everything we went through. There is a lot of emotion involved when someone in the family suffers a trauma no matter how big or small – not only for the victim of the trauma, but for their family as well.

Remember to be kind to each other, take a break, spend some time apart, find joint and personal hobbies/interests, encourage each other and don't judge.

Communicate – with each other and your professional help – and never give up hope.

Thank you for taking the time to read our story and I truly hope that some aspects are of benefit to you and yours as you navigate your own journey.

Alone we can do so little,
together we can do so much.

HELEN KELLER

Support

Do you, or does someone you know, need help?

GriefLine – Support for people experiencing loss or grief – griefline.org.au. Call 1300 845 745

MensLine Australia – A professional telephone and online counselling service offering support to Australian men, 24 hours/7 days a week, chat online or organise a video chat. Call 1300 78 99 78

eheadspace – Provides free online and telephone support and counselling to young people aged 12–25 and their families and friends. 9 am – 1 am AEST / 7 days a week, chat online or email. https://headspace.org.au

Beyond Blue – www.beyondblue.org.au

Lifeline – 24 hour telephone counselling service for people in crisis. Call 131 114

Mental Health Access Line (acute care) – 24 hour emergency phone service for people in acute psychiatric illness or distress. Leads to access to local public mental health services at local hospitals and emergency departments. Call 1800 011 511

Calm Harm – Resist or manage the urge to self harm

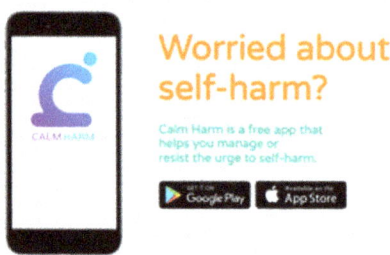

Move Mood – Helpful for depression and low mood

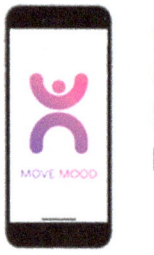
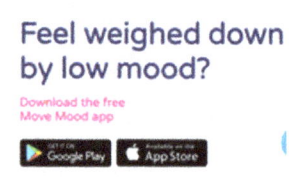

www.ingramcontent.com/pod-product-compliance
Lightning Source LLC
Chambersburg PA
CBHW051540010526
44107CB00064B/2799